Modern western science has shined an important light on the health and societal benefits of Tai Chi, but it often neglects its less tangible and poetic gifts—insights and guidance on how to navigate the sometimes complex and challenging human journey. Although I never had the opportunity to directly learn from Mr. Lui, I am deeply touched by the rich, practical, and often playful insights embodied in his sayings and borrowed quotes. And I am equally moved by the commitment and palpable gratitude of his students who assembled this lovely compendium of wisdom pearls into categories that allow the reader to feel as if they too can learn from their beloved teacher. A teacher's highest goal is to awaken in their students the same love and commitment to exploring Tai Chi as they experienced. I believe this book is a resounding endorsement of Mr. Lui's success and I recommend it to all.

—***Peter M. Wayne, Ph.D.,*** Bernard Osher Associate Professor of Medicine in the Field of Complementary and Integrative Medical Therapies, Harvard Medical School; Director, Osher Center for Integrative Health, Brigham and Women's Hospital and Harvard Medical School; author of *The Harvard Medical School Guide to Tai Chi*

Not many of us feel we are loved enough, or in quite the right way. We all feel deficient in Vitamin L (Love) sometimes. Mr. Lui's most needed teaching is that love is not something to be expected from others but something we find with others, generated among us when we learn to say yes, to yield, to sing, to help our friends excel.

—***Anne O'Byrne, Ph.D.,*** Professor of Philosophy, Stony Brook University, author of *Natality and Finitude* and *The Genocide Paradox*

These Spiritual Snacks are very rich in Vitamin L (Love). One is energized with the L Vitamin by every single word of this book. Mr. H. H. Lui found the means of expressing the powerful L Vitamin through the practice of tai chi. The overflow of Mr. Lui's Vitamin L emerges as an invitation to join him in the joy and harmony and fun that one encounters at the heart of the tai chi practice.

—***Jordi Torrent,*** Filmmaker, Duende Pictures; Former Media Educator at the United Nations

SPIRITUAL SNACKS

Teachings of H. H. Lui

SPIRITUAL SNACKS

Teachings of H. H. Lui

EDITED BY BARBARA ALDERSON

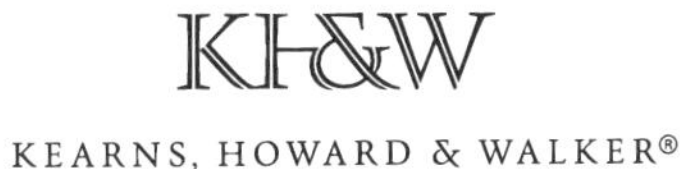

KEARNS, HOWARD & WALKER®

www.khwpublisher.com

Garden of Joy ©2011, cover painting by Gloria Matuszewski
www.gloriamatuszewski.com

Karen Ann Design, cover and book design

ISBN: 978-1-7354615-3-3

Dedicated to the memory of Hubert H. Lui
and the spirit of his teaching

The Way to a Happy Life

Keep your heart free from hate,
Your mind free from worry.
Live simply, expect little, and give much.[1]
Fill your life with Vitamin L (love).[2]
See beauty in the commonplace.[3]
Scatter sunshine.
Forget self, think of others.[1]
Regard all good deeds you do as ends,
Not means to an end.[4]
Do your job and claim no credit.[5]

[1] Norman Vincent Peale
[2] H. H. Lui
[3] Proverbial Wisdom
[4] Immanuel Kant, variant H. H. Lui
[5] Lao Tzu, trans. H. H. Lui

CONTENTS

INTRODUCTION

For almost thirty years, Hubert H. Lui taught the practice, spirit, and philosophy of tai chi, always emphasizing family, friendship, and community as the basis for a harmonious life. "Fill your life with Vitamin L (love)," he would say. This book, a tribute to a beloved teacher, is a compilation of Mr. Lui's sayings as drawn together by his students.

His style was noteworthy for its emphasis on encouragement with an overlay of humor. To urge openness, he would often say, "Don't be a cement head." For discipline, he might quip, "Don't fall in love with your bed." And joy, he said, "is found all along the way."

Mr. Lui, born Lui Hok Hoi in China in 1911, began studying tai chi in Hong Kong in 1953, continuing his studies in Chicago after immigrating to the United States. He began teaching tai chi in Chicago, where he founded and directed the tai chi program at the Dance Center of Columbia College Chicago from 1972 to 1979. Mr. Lui continued teaching until his death in 1995, holding classes and retreats first in Illinois, then in Michigan, Oregon, New York, and California.

After he and his wife, Elsie Lui, retired from their jobs in Chicago, they moved to San Francisco where they remained for the rest of their lives. From 1980 to 1995, Mr. Lui created and led an annual Tai Chi Friends Reunion in San Francisco, bringing together his students, and eventually their students, to learn and practice tai chi and to gather in friendship. The rest of the year, he stayed in contact with local and far-flung students through classes and correspondence, including what he called "Spiritual Snacks," one-page compilations he periodically shared of his ideas and related quotations.

In teaching movement, discipline, and the values of tai chi, Mr. Lui referenced many sources of wisdom. He found commonalities among traditional tai chi and Taoist sources, varied religious teachings, proverbial or folk wisdom, and the popular culture of his time.

Mr. Lui saw tai chi as a path to wisdom and a good life. He taught that we grow into wisdom as we live the tai chi spirit, and we grow into the good life through relationships with self, others, and nature. Lofty goals, but what do such goals mean in our daily lives?

For Mr. Lui, this meant bringing an open mind to see beyond ourselves, to appreciate the joy of the daily world in all its beauty, to be present in the moment, to understand that change is constant. We practice selflessness and humility, offer service to others, share our knowledge, and learn from the knowledge of other people and from nature. We develop friendships and relationships. We act with Vitamin L, Mr. Lui's prescription for love. Taking and giving Vitamin L is essential for wisdom, for a consummate tai chi life, and for fostering joy. This, he believed, and as many of his students can attest, allows us to live in harmony with ourselves, others, and nature.

Those who learned from Mr. Lui understand that tai chi and harmony require perseverance, focus, and dedication. Just as developing tai chi skills requires practice, so does developing our lives. As we practice harmony, friendship, and peace, we develop deeper harmony, friendship, and peace. We find joy all along the way.

This compendium assembles quotations and sayings Mr. Lui used in his tai chi classes and teachings. Although he taught these ideas through his tai chi, they are not restricted to any one discipline. These quotations, proverbial wisdoms, and maxims express waymarks toward the achievable harmonious life Mr. Lui believed was available to everyone. We hope they will inspire and guide you as they have inspired and guided us over the years.

EDITORIAL NOTE

The quotations in this book are drawn from the "Spiritual Snacks" flyers, Mr. Lui's tai chi diaries, student memories, and, unless otherwise indicated, Mr. Lui's translations from Chinese philosophy. While every effort has been made to accurately present Mr. Lui's words, quotations have been edited for clarity and for inclusivity.

All historic texts remain in their original form.

Insofar as verifiable, we have directly identified the source of quotations by their author.

We have used these citations for quotations more challenging to ascribe:

Anonymous: author is unknown

Attributed to: direct source could not be verified, but is often conjectured to be from a particular source

Proverbial Wisdom: ascribed to numerous sources

Tai Chi Maxim: ascribed to numerous tai chi sources

trans.: translated by a particular person

variant: modified from an original source, often by H. H. Lui

Chinese terms used in the quotations:

chi: intrinsic energy

chi gung: holistic Chinese exercise where chi is experienced more immediately than in the more challenging practice of tai chi chuan

jin: intrinsic energy combined with strength

Tao: the path or the way

tan tien: center of intrinsic energy, about 2-3 inches below the navel

tai chi chuan: holistic Chinese exercise and energy-cultivation system

yi: the will

yin yang: complementary opposites

OPEN MIND

Don't be a cement head!

We are born with two eyes, two ears, but only one mouth; therefore, we should look and listen twice as much as we speak.

—Proverbial Wisdom

Learn to live in harmony with nature, with ourselves, and with others.

—Proverbial Wisdom

Ego is the primary source of all our disasters and the cardinal obstacle to making friends and influencing people.

—H. H. Lui

Smash your ego into mashed potatoes.

—H. H. Lui

Don't be a cement head!

—H. H. Lui

Whatsoever you sow that you shall also reap.

—Galatians 6:7 (King James Bible), variant H. H. Lui

Commentary: You sow tai chi seed; you shall reap tai chi fruit. You serve tai chi well; tai chi serves you even better. Tai chi, as well as life, is exactly what you put in, no more, no less.

—H. H. Lui

A tree is known by its fruit.

—Matthew 12:33 (King James Bible), variant H. H. Lui

Commentary: If your heart has tai chi friends, your class, workshop, and friend circle will also have tai chi friends.

—H. H. Lui

Each day look at a beautiful picture,
Read a beautiful poem,
Listen to some beautiful music,
And, if possible, say some reasonable thing.

—Johann Wolfgang Goethe

The best and most beautiful things in the world cannot be seen or touched; they must be felt by the heart.

—Helen Keller

The greater your heart, the bigger your world.

—H. H. Lui

The world is full of beauty when your heart is full of love.

—Gaetano Donizetti

Nature is a silent teacher. When you have a problem, you don't have peace of mind, go to see nature. Go hiking. Go camp. Go see nature. Go for a walk in the woods. Go to the mountaintop. Very good!! Go walk on the sandy beach. You'll feel yourself small. Then you will enjoy peace of mind.

—H. H. Lui

People tire quickly of new discoveries and inventions, but never of the beauty and wonder of nature.

—Proverbial Wisdom

Tai chi tells the peacemaker, "Before trying to make peace throughout the world, first make peace within yourself."

—H. H. Lui

There is no way to peace. Peace is the way.

—A. J. Muste

Think with the learned, and speak with the vulgar.

—George Berkeley

And what is a weed? A plant whose virtues have not been discovered.

—Ralph Waldo Emerson

Everybody is ignorant only on different subjects.

—Will Rogers

If you sit at the bottom of a well
and look at the sky from inside,
however you twist your neck,
your view cannot be wide.

—Proverbial Wisdom

Advice is seldom welcome, and those who want it the most like it the least.

—Lord Chesterfield

On the Tao, life seeks you. Life becomes easy, you exert very little effort and accomplish a lot. Deviating from or against the Tao, you seek life. Life becomes difficult. You exert a lot of effort and accomplish very little.

—H. H. Lui

Life makes fun of you!

—Proverbial Wisdom

Upon the great sea of spirit, there is room for every sail. In the limitless sky of truth, there is room for every wing.

—Mirza Ahmad Sohrab

Commentary: Tai chi teaches us to have an open mind and a big heart. Tolerance is the word.

—H. H. Lui

GROWTH

On the Tao, things grow.

To recognize our knowledge as ignorance,
This is noble insight.
To regard our ignorance as knowledge,
This is mental sickness.

—Lao Tzu, trans. John C. H. Wu

Commentary: To realize our ignorance is the first step toward knowledge. Humility is the word.

—H. H. Lui

Know Thyself.

—Proverbial Wisdom

Commentary: We must learn to recognize our own weaknesses. When we are truly humble, we enjoy peace of mind.

—H. H. Lui

I-center, egoism, selfishness, and cement-headedness are no friends to truth and wisdom and are the cardinal obstacles to our tai chi progress and our personal growth.

—H. H. Lui

Tai chi must be born out of ourselves in the process of manifesting the truth, the goodness and the beauty of nature; it must be born out of the emotion and the life experiences of our time; it must be ever growing and it must be always fresh.

—H. H. Lui

What you are going to be, you are now becoming.

—Attributed to Carl R. Rogers

Once the teacher has planted the seed, it is up to the student to take care of it and help it grow.

—Proverbial Wisdom

We are beset with great troubles because we are conscious of self. If we are selfless, what trouble can we have? Hence self is the primary source of all our calamities.

—H. H. Lui

If you are patient in one moment of anger, you will escape 100 days of sorrow.

—Chinese Proverb

If you make a mistake and correct it, no mistake.

—H. H. Lui

No one can force you to do good; you have to choose to do good.

—Proverbial Wisdom

Do not let your mouth issue checks that your heart cannot cash.

—Proverbial Wisdom

An exaggeration is a truth that has lost its temper.

—Kahlil Gibran

You can do what you want, but you pay for it.

—Proverbial Wisdom

One who has a beautiful soul always has some beautiful things to say, but one who says beautiful things does not necessarily have a beautiful soul.

—Proverbial Wisdom

Slow me down, Lord, and inspire me to send my roots deep into the soil of life's enduring values that I may grow toward the stars of my greater destiny.

—Attributed to Orin L. Crain

The older you are the happier you are. When you get older, you lose more devils and you gain more angels.

—H. H. Lui

Get old too quick, get smart too late.

—Dutch Proverb

Tai chi friends may come and go, but tai chi is everlasting. Tai chi behavior involves both give and take, input and output, learning and teaching, receiving and sharing, listening to the positive comments and the negative comments. In fact, tai chi learning encompasses all the adversities that make you grow faster and healthier. We should learn to meet all the challenges and welcome them with open arms, open mind, and open heart.

—H. H. Lui

The mind grows by what it feeds on.

—Josiah Gilbert Holland

Commentary: If you feed on "tai chi for peace and harmony," your mind will grow toward the direction of peace and harmony.

—H. H. Lui

If you live by public opinion, you'll never be rich;
if you live with nature, you'll never be poor.

—Epicurus, quoted by Seneca, variant H. H. Lui

The Path (Tao) may not be left for an instant;
if it could be left, it would not be the Path (Tao).

—Confucius, variant H. H. Lui

On the Tao, things grow. Deviate from the Tao and things stand still. Against the Tao things decline.

—H. H. Lui

WATER WISDOM

*Only the law of changeability
does not change.*

When one gets into trouble, one must change one's way to deal with the situation. Change is the road to solution.

—*I Ching, trans. H. H. Lui*

Have water wisdom, not a cement head.

—*H. H. Lui*

We often grow more by bending with the wind than by standing in rigid defiance.

—*Proverbial Wisdom*

Commentary: This appears to be the proper way of learning tai chi and making friends. Yielding is the word!

—*H. H. Lui*

When you are in the stage of "Seeking the Truth, the Water Wisdom," like seeking peace of mind, you have to move around, jumping from one place to another with your body, mind, and spirit like a busy bee. As a result, you are not at home in body, mind, and spirit, cannot quietly sit down or settle down, and we call this "pointed butt."

On the other hand, after you have found the Truth, the Water Wisdom, you no longer run, drive, or fly from one place to another, aimless as a destination-less "blind-headed fly." You have found your home and are able to settle down peacefully at home, home sweet home in body, mind, and spirit. You have time to enjoy life and choose to´ do the things you like.

You have your schedule, you have your plan and you are no longer being pushed around by temptations or others and you lose desire or interest in all or any kind of vanity, popularity, competition, argument, or being No. 1. You do the things that enrich your life and enjoy peace of mind and plentiful life. And we style this period of lifetime as "flat butt," and we enjoy life.

—H. H. Lui

Don't be a pointy butt!

—H. H. Lui

I can't change the direction of the wind, but I can adjust my sails to always reach my destination.

—Jimmy Dean

When the horse is dead, get off and walk.

—Proverbial Wisdom

The birds of worry and care fly above your head, this you cannot change. If they build nests in your hair, this you can prevent.

—Proverbial Wisdom

One who builds a house on the water's edge is the first to see the light of the moon.

—Proverbial Wisdom

When a plant is living, it is soft and tender.
When it is dead, it becomes withered and dry.

Hence, the hard and rigid belongs to the company
of the dead:
The soft and supple belongs to the company of
the living.

Therefore, a mighty army tends to fall by its own
weight,
Just as dry wood is ready for the ax.

The mighty and great will be laid low;
The humble and weak will be exalted.

—Lao Tzu, trans. John C. H. Wu

Bamboo:

1. rooted and flexible
2. hollow, empty—humble
3. green—purity of nature
4. segmental—never stretches too far or falls too short

Be like the bamboo.

—H. H. Lui

To yield is to be preserved whole;
To be bent is to become straight;
To be hollow is to be filled;
To be tattered is to be renewed;[1]
To have little is to gain;
To have much is to be confused.[2]

—[1] Lao Tzu, trans. Lin Yutang
—[2] Lao Tzu, trans. H. H. Lui

Commentary: Lao Tzu observed that to have too much (too many diverse desires and interests) is to be confused. To have little (to be single-minded) is to gain.

—H. H. Lui

Few things under heaven are as instructive as the lessons of Silence, or as beneficial as the fruits of Non-Ado.

—Lao Tzu, trans. John C. H. Wu

Commentary: Do nothing and nothing is undone.

—Lao Tzu, trans. H. H. Lui

The sage does the job and claims no credit.

—Lao Tzu, trans. H. H. Lui

How does the sea become the king of all streams?
Because it lies lower than they!
Hence, it is the king of all streams.

—Lao Tzu, trans. John C. H. Wu

Commentary: Humble down yourself. Humility is the word.

—H. H. Lui

Angels can fly because they can take themselves lightly.

—G. K. Chesterton

I don't worry about not being recognized; I worry that I'm not worthy to be recognized.

—Proverbial Wisdom

Always remember that life is like a coin which has two sides: If you love the rainbow, you must also love the rain; if you love the rose, you must also love the thorn.

—Proverbial Wisdom

For a whirlwind does not last a whole morning,
Nor does a sudden shower last a whole day.

—Lao Tzu, trans. John C. H. Wu

Serenity is not freedom from the storm, but peace amid the storm.

—Proverbial Wisdom

Commentary: When we learn tai chi, we learn true serenity.

—H. H. Lui

Be like the lotus, a flower that grows in muddy water yet remains pure and lives immaculately above it.

—Proverbial Wisdom

Under heaven all things change and only the law of changeability does not change.

—H. H. Lui

JOY

Happiness is found all along the way,
not at the end of the way.

Where there is love, there is peace.
Where there is peace, there is harmony.
Where there is harmony, there is growth.
Where there is growth, there is joy! Joy! Joy!

—H. H. Lui

On the Tao, things turn out better than expected.

—H. H. Lui

Keep a green tree in your heart and a singing bird will come.

—Chinese Proverb, trans. H. H. Lui

I slept and dreamed that life was joy,
I awoke and saw that life was duty,
I acted and beheld that duty was joy.

—Rabindranath Tagore

The Joy is in the doing. It is
Found all along the way.
Not at the end of the way.
This is the Art of Life.

—H. H. Lui

"Time flies like an arrow through space."
Enjoy it all the way!

—H. H. Lui, quotation Anonymous

I love to look at the world and life from the beautiful side and see it with a telescope, not a microscope.

—H. H. Lui

You see the flower and the tree and the bird. All the way. You enjoy it. This is the Art of Life. You must learn it. You enjoy it all. The whole world is your material, your university. Every minute is abundant life.

—H. H. Lui

Vitamin L therapy:
Where there is love, there is beauty. Where there is beauty, there is joy.

—H. H. Lui

Laugh therapy:
Three laughs a day drives the doctors away! Laughter conserves energy. It is positive thinking in action!

—H. H. Lui

In a 1,000 mile journey every step is an end; hence, you enjoy every step. In practicing tai chi, you treat every movement as an end, not as a means to an end, so you are able to enjoy tai chi all the way.

—H. H. Lui

A tai chi body is light and lightness leads to nimbleness and nimbleness leads to agility and agility leads to movement and movement leads to action and action leads to development and development leads to progress and progress leads to J-O-Y!

—H. H. Lui

No lousy moments!

—H. H. Lui

A Buddhist tale:
One of the students asked the teacher how to find happiness.

The teacher replied, "The secret is in an iron box. I will give you the key to the box. The box is on a mountaintop. You must climb three hours to the mountaintop, open the iron box, and there you will find the secret.

The student awoke the next day and walked and walked. Walk. Walk. Walk. Walk like hell! All the while, the student was thinking "the secret, the secret, the secret."

At last, the exhausted student arrived at the top of the mountain, found the box, and opened it. On a piece of paper was printed: "Happiness is found all along the way, not at the end of the way."

—As told by H. H. Lui

In tai chi as in life, joy is not found at the end of the road, but all the way along the road. You enjoy the means as much as the end. In fact, tai chi practice is an end in itself and not a means to an end.

—H. H. Lui

TOGETHERNESS

Making friends is the high art of life.

Making friends is the high art of life. No friends, no life; no good friends, no good life; no abundant friends, no abundant life.

To make friends:

1. Practice the art of yielding.
2. Learn to sing along with your friends.
3. Don't be a victim of negativism. Don't get in the habit of saying "no" when others say "yes," or when others say "no," you say "yes."
4. Don't let yourself outsmart others. If you want to make friends, let others excel more than you; if you want to make enemies, let yourself excel over others.

The law of life is as simple as that.

—H. H. Lui

Knowledge breeds knowledge, friendship breeds friendship, outgoing communications attract incoming communications, like the circular tai chi movement without end.

—H. H. Lui

In our tai chi family, there is no east or west. In it, no this school or that school but one great fellowship of love!

—H. H. Lui

In tai chi, we don't struggle within ourselves or with others but rather act within ourselves and with others. Thus, in the tai chi life, it is easy to make friends.

—H. H. Lui

Love is the master that opens up the gate to happiness.

—Oliver Wendell Holmes

Commentary: Like the stars and the moon illuminate the heavens, we tai chi friends light up each other's lives.

—H. H. Lui

Tai chi is an exercise of love, peace, harmony, and joy. It adds years to your life (longevity) and life to your years (abundant life). How good and pleasant it is for our tai chi friends to practice together, breakfast together, learn together, have fun and fellowship together, and grow together in harmony and in unity.

—H. H. Lui

A marriage is a polarity, not a duality. It is a yin yang harmony oneness. Loving partners supplement each other and attract but do not repel each other.

—H. H. Lui

Each couple representing a "harmonious one" is better prepared to share with others, to contribute to the happiness of others, and to enjoy a "community harmony openness." Indeed, an enduring, endurable, and happy family is a "we-centered," not an "I-centered," family.

—H. H. Lui

Family first.

—Proverbial Wisdom

In life, your family should be first, your job second, and practicing tai chi third.

—H. H. Lui

Harmony is greater than truth.

—H. H. Lui

The three great harmonies: people, location, weather. The most important? People.

—H. H. Lui

Humanitarianism consists in never sacrificing a human being to a purpose.

—Attributed to Albert Schweitzer

Heaven lasts long, and Earth abides.
What is the secret of their durability?
Is it not because they do not live for themselves
That they can live so long?

—Lao Tzu, trans. John C. H. Wu

Commentary: Selflessness is the word.

—H. H. Lui

Those who bring sunshine to the lives of others cannot keep it from themselves.

—James M. Barrie

There is no better exercise for the heart than bending down and lifting someone up.

—John Andrew Holmes

Always yield to the weakest member of the group. If your friend can't walk very fast, slow down your pace.

—H. H. Lui

If I can walk ten miles and my spouse can walk five miles, walk five miles and take a taxi. How nice!

—H. H. Lui

Tai chi serves not only to develop your chi, but to direct your chi to proper uses for the benefit of others.

—H. H. Lui

Do unto others as though you were the others.

—Luke 6:31 (King James Bible), variant

The time is always right to do what is right.

—Dr. Martin Luther King, Jr.

To handle yourself, use your head, to handle others, use your heart.

—Attributed to Eleanor Roosevelt

On making decisions:

1. If you make decisions while you are off-center and emotionally upset, you will regret it in later days. If you make decisions while you are centered and rationally calm, you will enjoy peace of mind all the way.
2. If you make decisions with a group attitude and a community-centered interest, you will always have company and support. If you make decisions without a group attitude and with only an individual-centered interest, you will always be alone and fighting the battle single-handedly.

—H. H. Lui

The joy is in the sharing, particularly sharing the words of truth and wisdom.

—H. H. Lui

Love (Vitamin L) is the fuel (fire, high chi) to cook a warm heart. Enthusiasm is the propeller to inspire following the way of Tao, of rightness.

—H. H. Lui

Remember: Vitamin L (love) and Vitamin E (enthusiasm) are the two most important vitamins to nourish a successful and happy life. With "L" and "E," a difficult task becomes an easy job; without "L" and "E," an easy job becomes a difficult task. True in tai chi!

—H. H. Lui

Vitamin L (love) is the vitamin of vitamins. It is the basic virtue needed "to make friends and influence people."

—H. H. Lui, quotation Dale Carnegie, variant H. H. Lui

Love unites, opinion divides.

—H. H. Lui

Tai chi is the work of love; there is no discord in love: the love within the tai chi practitioner's self, between the self and others and between the practitioner and the universe. To love is to conserve energy.

—H. H. Lui

There is no remedy for a lack of Vitamin L (love) but to take more Vitamin L.

—H. H. Lui

Those who love most spend most; those who hoard most lose much.

—Lao Tzu, trans. H. H. Lui

Commentary: If your friend invites you for a cup of coffee, invite them for lunch; if they invite you for lunch, take them to dinner.

—H. H. Lui

Vitamin L (love) in action and community, participation, presence, and humility. Vitamin L and high chi—because there is no other way.

—H. H. Lui

Show your love. Show your Vitamin L. You say "I love people. I love humanity." Your humanity must extend beyond your own skin. Loving without giving is NOTHING! It is a lazy person's philosophy, a lazy person's exercise, a lazy person's religion.

—H. H. Lui

As the sun illuminates the stars in heaven, so our tai chi friends illuminate each other on earth!

—H. H. Lui

Don't be a "tai chi holic" or any "holic." In good times, share your good fortune with others. In bad times others will help you to jump over the hurdle. You need not fight the battle single-handedly. You will not be alone! Thus, selfishness has no place in a happy life.

—H. H. Lui

The true people see the common nature among things in the universe and discard all their differences.

—Attributed to Chuang Tzu, trans. H. H. Lui

PERSEVERANCE

You must have follow-through spirit.

NPNB PHD for tai chi success.
No Practice, No Breakfast!

Patience—Perseverance,
Humility—Humanity,
Dedication—Determination,
For there is no other way.

—H. H. Lui

As a bird needs two wings to fly, a tai chi practitioner needs two "tions" to learn, inspiration and perspiration: inspiration from the teacher and perspiration from the student. One hand cannot clap.

—H. H. Lui

"A song is not a song unless you sing it." Tai chi is not tai chi unless you practice it—practice not only the form or movement but the philosophy behind it.

—H. H. Lui, quotation Oscar Hammerstein II

Tai chi is not a weekend or do-as-you-please commitment. In order to reap full benefits, one must practice daily. "If you miss one day, you know it. If you miss two days, your teacher knows it. If you miss three days, the whole world knows it." NPNB-NPNB-NPNB (No Practice, No Breakfast)

—H. H. Lui, quotation Franz Liszt, variant H. H. Lui

Practice, practice, practice! There is no other way.

—H. H. Lui

To get to the top of an oak tree, you can sit on an acorn and wait for the tree to grow or find an oak tree and climb.

—Kemmons Wilson, variant H. H. Lui

Commentary: In tai chi, we climb!

—H. H. Lui

A journey of a thousand miles starts with a single step.

—Lao Tzu, trans. H. H. Lui

A ship in a harbor is safe, but that is not what ships were built for.

—John A. Shedd

Don't fall in love with your bed!

—H. H. Lui

The world belongs to the energetic.

—Ralph Waldo Emerson

Be on time! Punctuality is very important. It shows that your mind is in control of your body.

—H. H. Lui

The four most important things in life:

1. be on time,
2. pay attention,
3. tell the truth, and
4. don't be attached to the consequence of telling the truth.

—H. H. Lui

Draw a straight line from your tan tien to your destination in order to get there efficiently and on time.

—H. H. Lui

If all the year were playing holidays, to sport would be as tedious as to work.

—Shakespeare, Henry IV, Part 1

Commentary: There is no such problem in tai chi life. In tai chi work while you work, play while you play; there involves a harmonious interplaying of yin and yang, of a well-balanced input and output of your energy.

—H. H. Lui

High energy acts fast.

—H. H. Lui

Talk less, move more.

—H. H. Lui

Those who talk by yard, but act by inch, should be kicked by foot.

—Anonymous

Failing to prepare is preparing to fail.

—Proverbial Wisdom

Margin theory:
Always allow an extra 15 minutes in case of a problem.

—H. H. Lui

Leave a 15-minute margin, so you have time to visit with friends and neighbors you may meet along the way to your destination and not be in a rush.

—H. H. Lui

When traveling, carry a light suitcase and a heavy wallet.

—H. H. Lui

To know when you have enough is to be immune
from disgrace.
To know when to stop is to be preserved from perils.
Only thus can you endure long.

—Lao Tzu, trans. John C. H. Wu

Do the thing you hate. That is the sign of a strong person. Weak people do only the easy things.

—Dante Benedetti

It is not doing the things we like to do, but liking the things we have to do that make life blessed.

—Attributed to Johann Wolfgang Goethe

Never quit but rather welcome any and all challenges in life. "Do the things you hate," not the things you like, as long as they make your life blessed. Be optimistic and laugh your troubles away. Positive thinking conserves energy, and makes you truly strong.

—H. H. Lui

To me, adversity is but an inspiration.

—H. H. Lui

The path of least resistance:
Act without action; work without effort.
Taste without savoring.
Magnify the small; increase the few.
Repay ill will with kindness.
Plan the difficult when it is easy;
Handle the big when it is small.
The world's hardest work begins when it is easy;
The world's largest effort begins when it is small.
Evolved individuals, finally, take no great action,
And in that way the great is achieved.
Those who commit easily, inspire little trust.
How easy to inspire hardness!
Therefore evolved individuals view all as difficult.
Finally they have no difficulty!

—Lao Tzu, trans. H. H. Lui

You must have follow-through spirit.

—H. H. Lui

LEARNING & TEACHING

The students make the master
and not the other way around.

If you want to reap the utmost from the Tai Chi Friends Reunion or any learning experience, lend me your ears:

1. Bring an empty cup, not a full cup, to the class. In tai chi, it is only the humble who can learn.
2. Bring two ears to the class. One ear to listen to favorable or positive comments about you, the other ear to listen to unfavorable or negative comments about you. While you should have a thankful heart to appreciate all the good words, you also should have an open mind to welcome all criticisms. In fact, it is criticism that makes you grow strong. Adversity is the most effective education.
3. Bring no conclusions to the class. Foregone conclusions, arbitrary predetermination, obstinacy, and egotism are the cardinal obstacles to personal growth. An I-center is an isolated center. To realize our ignorance is the first step to tai chi wisdom.

—H. H. Lui

I love my teacher, but I love the truth more.

—Aristotle, variant

I hear and I forget,
I see and I cannot remember,
I do and I understand.

—Xunzi, variant

If a teacher sounds too mystical, find another one. If a teacher is too commercial, find another one. If a teacher loves publicity too much, find another one. If a teacher is not interested in answering any sensible question, find another one. If a teacher appears to be at a lower energy level than the students, find another one. If a teacher regards their own master as a god and their teaching entirely flaw free, find another one. If a teacher does not practice what is taught—a poor personal witness—find another one.

—H. H. Lui

A good leader is a good follower.

—Proverbial Wisdom

Only when you have can you give;
only when you know can you teach.

—H. H. Lui

A wise person learns more from a fool than a fool learns from a wise person.

—Cato the Elder

Professor Albert Einstein was asked what he considered the best formula for success in life.

"If A is success in life," he replied, "I should say the formula is A=X+Y+Z, X being work and Y being play."

"And what," I asked, "is Z?"

"That," he answered, "is keeping your mouth shut."

—S. J. Woolf

The wise speak because they have something to say; the fools because they have to say something.

—Proverbial Wisdom

The learned Fool writes his Nonsense in better Language than the unlearned; but still 'tis Nonsense.

—Benjamin Franklin

April 1st is the day upon which we are reminded of what we are the other 364.

—Mark Twain

Those who know and know they know
are wise; follow them.
Those who know and know not they know
are asleep; wake them.
Those who know not and know they know not
are children; teach them.
Those who know not, and know not they know not
are fools; shun them.

—Proverbial Wisdom

The function of tai chi education consists of not only the art of developing chi but also the art of using that chi in the pursuit of goodness, such as: fill yourself with love, scatter sunshine, live for others, harmonize with heaven and earth, know yourself, and conquer yourself. Then witness peace.

—H. H. Lui

In teaching tai chi, you must be a good personal witness of the tai chi way of life and spirit (very challenging) or else your words carry no weight. Teachers and students are mutually inspiring; good teachers usually attract good students and good students usually bring out teachers' good teaching methods and good teaching material.

—H. H. Lui

In order to be a successful learner, one must embrace three "hearts" or "minds": a heart of determination, a heart of faith, and a heart of constancy.

—Tai Chi Maxim, variant H. H. Lui

What is well planted cannot be uprooted.
What is well embraced cannot slip away.

—Lao Tzu, trans. John C. H. Wu

Commentary: If you treat tai chi like a motel, you will be treated as a guest; if you treat it like a home, you will be embraced like family.

—H. H. Lui

Never worship your teacher or any teacher as if a god. Never fall in love with your own way of doing tai chi or with your own way of life.

—H. H. Lui

Nothing in tai chi chuan is so mystical that you cannot understand it yourself with common sense and daily practice.

—H. H. Lui

There is no graduation from the tai chi university. The more you learn, the less you know. Tai chi is like the horizon: the nearer you approach it, the farther it recedes.

—H. H. Lui

The end of the tai chi workshop is the beginning of tai chi.

—H. H. Lui

Practice tai chi for ten years, then tell me if you like it.

—H. H. Lui

Take deeper tai chi root, bear better tai chi fruit with ten times return! If you serve tai chi diligently and faithfully, tai chi serves you even better!

—H. H. Lui

When I meet someone, I judge them. If they know more than me, I learn from them. If they know less than me, I teach them.

—H. H. Lui

The students make the master and not the other way around.

—H. H. Lui

You can teach what you know.

—H. H. Lui to Shizu Lofton

If I know ten things, I will teach you all ten. I will not teach just eight and keep two to myself so I will know more than you. I will teach you all ten and then I will know eleven.

—H. H. Lui

The first time you repeat something I say, you can attribute it to me; the second time, it's yours.

—H. H. Lui

When a tai chi practitioner humbly and seriously asks to learn one secret, the teacher should be more than happy to share two. Knowledge breeds knowledge.

—H. H. Lui

Tai chi is a universal light, an eternal truth. It is great; so great that no one individual, one family, one organization, or one country can house it. Tai chi is heaven's gift and nobody can own it or should treat it as personal property. Thus, everyone is entitled to learn it and everyone is entitled to teach it. I must not be stingy in teaching. I must teach generously.

—H. H. Lui

MOVEMENT

When you are in perfect harmony,
each movement becomes music.

The 7 essentials of tai chi practice:

1. Humble yourself down, lower and lower.
2. Let the chi freely flow through the entire body, slower and slower.
3. Practice and practice makes perfect. Repeat a single movement 1,000 times.
4. Be gradual, move inch by inch, no jerks, no sudden actions, and no sharp angles.
5. Round and round, "Merry Go Round." All movements are spirals in the form of circles, arches, or waves.
6. Refuse to give up. NPNB (No Practice, No Breakfast) is a daily must.
7. Do tai chi with your heart. Tai chi has life and it can grow and thrive.

—H. H. Lui

Isadora Duncan, the pioneer of modern dance, observed that one of the characteristics of "true dance" is its "wave movement." She said, "All movements in nature seem to me to have as their ground plan the law of wave movement … all energy expresses itself through this wave movement … all free natural movements conform to the law of wave movement. It is the alternative attraction and resistance of the law of gravity that causes this wave movement."

In tai chi, the practitioner moves up and down, forward and back, advances and retreats, yields and bounces back, indicating the two opposite cosmic forces interplaying with each other. If this interplay is in perfect harmony, the things involved will grow. When moving up, advancing, bouncing back, you release energy and you exhale. On the contrary, when moving down, retreating, yielding, you store energy and you inhale. At this moment you are drawing your body along with the center of gravity. The interplay of these two opposite forces, yin (storing energy movement) and yang (releasing energy movement) constitutes the wave or circular movement.

It is this wave or circular movement that makes the continuity of tai chi movement possible, and it is the continuous movement that helps the practitioner develop energy and high chi, the very goal of tai chi practice.

—H. H. Lui

Like all movements in nature, all tai chi movements must follow the law of wave movement, because nothing that endures in nature suggests jerks, sharp angles, breaks, or sudden action. Thus, in tai chi continuous and smooth movement and the free flowing of chi are essential.

—H. H. Lui

Poised like a scale, move like a wheel.

—Wang Chung-Yueh

Stages of training:
Learn the tai chi rules (the way of governing the tai chi movements). Be familiar with the rules (through diligent practice). Digest the rules (through deep study), and finally spiritualize the rules. Then you are free from the rules and not imprisoned by them, yet you do not deviate from the basic spirit of the rules.

—Tai Chi Maxim, variant H. H. Lui

Tai chi is not a race. Move at the pace of your breath and breathe deep.

—H. H. Lui

First move your body with your physical force, then with your chi (intrinsic energy), and then with your will (mind in action) and, finally, in the most advanced stage, move with your spirit. At this stage, you will practice tai chi free from the form and are no longer imprisoned by it—you are a real master.

—H. H. Lui

Don't be a victim of double weightedness. "You cannot blow and swallow at the same time." You cannot do the horse stance on two sailing boats.

—H. H. Lui, quotation Proverbial Wisdom

In tai chi, only when your movements are in tune with the rhythm of breathing can your movement be swift and active, just as the flowing object must be in oneness with the water current—the chi current.

—H. H. Lui

Rhythm in tai chi movement is of cardinal importance. In tai chi, the rhythm in movement is in harmony with the rhythm of the breathing which reflects the rhythm of the pulsation of the earth as one feels it. The rhythm in tai chi is the yin yang in action.

—H. H. Lui

Form efficiency:
In tai chi, the form and its function are integrated like other things in nature. The whole is greater than the sum of the parts, as with the structure of a bird or of the human body or the five fingers forming a fist.

—H. H. Lui

Paying too much attention or over focusing on movement or energy tends to cause suffering from tension and blocks the free flowing of energy.

—H. H. Lui

To move effortlessly, you must be relaxed throughout your whole self, most notably in your mind.

—H. H. Lui

Only when one can be extremely pliable and soft can one be extremely firm and hard.

—Wang Chung-Yueh

When your movement is hard, it must not be sluggish. When your movement is soft, it must not be loose. In quietude your movement is as still as the Tai Shan mountain. In motion your movement is as dynamic as a swimming dragon. The spiral energy is layer after layer without end. The circular movement is circle within circle and change after change in every area. This is the amazing essence of the way of tai chi chuan.

—H. H. Lui

Continuity in movement is a must in tai chi. Whenever the movement appears to discontinue, the jin (intrinsic energy combined with strength) still continues; whenever the jin appears to discontinue, the yi (the will) still continues; and whenever the yi appears to discontinue, the spirit still continues. Thus, the movement is always sustained by the spirit—the number one boss in tai chi movement.

—H. H. Lui

There is meaning and life in every one of your tai chi movements.

—H. H. Lui

Rootedness develops a heavy lower body and a light upper body (iron legs, paper head). Centeredness leads to a posture with central equilibrium (balance and steadiness).

—H. H. Lui

Sink your energy; you will enjoy a paper head (light upper body) and an iron leg (firm lower body).

—H. H. Lui

Sink low, kick high!

—Bradford C. Bennett

Lower and lower, slower and slower, better and better, better and better.

—*H. H. Lui*

Tai chi movement must be one with the movement which runs through the universe. The flowing of the chi current of the body must be in tune with the flowing of the chi current in the universe.

—*H. H. Lui*

When you are in perfect harmony, each movement becomes music.

—*H. H. Lui*

Every movement in tai chi exists primarily in nature. To do tai chi is to glorify the virtue of nature rather than to express one's self.

—*H. H. Lui*

In tai chi, the four limbs resemble the rim of the wheel and the center of the body (lower tan tien) is the hub. When you release your energy through the four limbs from the center as if opening an umbrella ("singing in the rain") with energy, your umbrella will naturally be fully stretched to its extremity (unless you deliberately direct your energy otherwise), and balance and centeredness are the result as a matter of course.

—H. H. Lui

In tai chi, no part works like hell, no part takes a vacation.

—H. H. Lui

The common nature and feature of all schools are that the ultimate goals of tai chi are emptiness and calmness. The basics are proper body position and the right way of movement, plus relaxation of both body and mind, sinking the chi, lightness, and nimbleness of the body.

—H. H. Lui

Through proper tai chi practice one will become inseparably a part of the great divine rhythm of the universe, and this harmony between self and the center of being will result as a matter of course in harmonious living.

—H. H. Lui

Tai chi is a total philosophy. It is not only a philosophy for physical health, it is also a philosophy for holistic health, a sound body, mind, and spirit. It regards all parts of the body, the mind, and the spirit as one integrated organic unit, not isolated from one another. If one part of the self moves, all parts of the self must move and move in harmony. I must check constantly if I am setting a good example.

—H. H. Lui

TAI CHI

Tai chi must be born out of ourselves.

The song of tai chi is a new song and is also an old song; it is a song composed for the classroom, also for the great society. It is a living philosophy; it is a way of life. It is a song of yielding, a song of humility, and a song of selflessness. It is a song of love and harmony and of inner peace and joy. It is a song of non-striving, of non-competition, and of non-violence. It is a song of "knowing ourselves rather than others and conquering ourselves rather than others." It is a song of "to benefit not to harm and to do our job, but compete with no one." It is a song which everybody can know, but not everybody can sing. To sing it is to practice it, to practice it in one's entire daily living.

—H. H. Lui, quotations Lao Tzu, trans. H. H. Lui

The true meaning of tai chi chuan:

1. Tai chi chuan has no form nor shape. It is not attached to any pattern.
2. The body is filled with chi and the individual chi is at one with the universal chi. Thus, there is no separation between the internal and external.
3. Your body disregards all the tangible and earthly things and moves in accordance with the law of nature.
4. Your body resembles a suspended bell in the mountains. It can move easily, smoothly, and swiftly in any direction.
5. You move naturally and effortlessly. Never exert yourself or go to the extreme.
6. When your mind relaxes, your spirit becomes alive. Only when your mind is relaxed can your spirit become active.
7. The natural power guided by your spirit is unlimited. It can move the mountains and turn over the seas.
8. In short, follow nature and stand up with heaven!

—H. H. Lui

Tai chi is a growing art. A true tai chi practitioner manages to expand awareness not only of the self, but also of a deeper and greater universal source common to all, much more beautiful than the individual self. The movements not only mirror all the natural things, but also all the actions of people in their relation to the universe. Thus, a true tai chi practitioner is a faithful witness to the truth, goodness, and beauty of nature.

—H. H. Lui

Tai Chi is for peace and for harmony. It seeks peace and harmony within ourselves and with others, and teaches us to expand our good energy toward others and to live for others—unselfishness is the word! The world is one!

—H. H. Lui

Tai chi is a bridge, not a wall. It serves to unite not to divide people. It unites body, mind, and spirit.

—H. H. Lui

In practicing tai chi, you don't use your hands or body, but you use your soul. Only thus can you feel heaven and people are one.

—H. H. Lui

Tai chi consists of three Hs, three Ls, and three usages:

Three Hs:

Hand (body)
Head (mind)
Heart (spirit)

Three Ls:

Loving (heart)
Learning (mind)
Living (body)

Three usages:

Use your Heart to Love.
Use your Mind to Think.
Use your Body to Practice.

—H. H. Lui

Tai chi philosophy is the soul and spirit of the forms of tai chi chuan. There can be no growth or depth in tai chi without philosophy.

—H. H. Lui

Tai chi means nothing to you unless you are in it—being a personal witness.

—H. H. Lui

They who know the truth are not equal to those who love it, and they who love it are not equal to those who delight in it.

—Confucius

Commentary: Those who know tai chi are not equal to those who love tai chi, and those who love tai chi are not equal to those who find joy in practicing tai chi.

—H. H. Lui

I keep the energy flowing and avoid doing anything that may block the free passage of chi, such as sudden jerks or partial body movements or movements that have corners or sharp angles. Of course, the mental current should flow freely, too. The mind, the energy, and the body should be the same thing, working together harmoniously for the same goal.

—H. H. Lui

There is interplay between tai chi movement and the practitioner's inner feeling, each developing out of the other and each serving as an impulse initiating and influencing the other. These are mutually growing and mutually arising.

—H. H. Lui

Tai chi will change your life.

—H. H. Lui

The kind of movement you practice develops a like-kind of chi and that kind of chi develops a like-kind of personality. If you execute your tai chi form in a peaceful, patient, gentle, continuous, and harmonious way, you will develop a similar personality; to the contrary, if you move in a violent, impatient, rough, jerky, and conflicted way, you will naturally develop a similar personality.

—H. H. Lui

Tai chi will make a young person feel old and an old person feel young.

—H. H. Lui

The law of increasing returns:
The more you practice tai chi, the younger you feel and the stronger you become.

—H. H. Lui

Before the study of tai chi, the body is like water. After studying tai chi for some time, the body is like warm water. Studying tai chi for a long time, the body is like hot water. After studying tai chi for a very long time (say 10-20 years) and having done it in the most proper way, the hot water transforms to steam, i.e., chi, then high chi. In this stage you enjoy a sense of lightness of both your mind and body and you feel more secure and have peace of mind.

—H. H. Lui

Tai chi movement without chi resembles a sail without wind, a boat without steam, water without current, words without deed, and tai chi harmony without tai chi friends. Without chi nothing can be accomplished.

—H. H. Lui

When your body is filled with chi, you naturally enjoy a sense of lightness in your movement.

—H. H. Lui

Tai chi education and practice is the function of an organism, not an organization! It's living and growing. Form without spirit is a dead form.

—H. H. Lui

The fine arts once divorcing themselves from truth are quite certain to fall mad if they do not die.

—Thomas Carlyle

Commentary: Tai chi chuan once divorcing itself from Tao (living philosophy of peace and harmony) is quite certain to fall into a fighting art or some sort of senseless exercise.

—H. H. Lui

The nature of tai chi:
A child is born and gifted with a tai chi body and a tai chi mind. Its bones and sinews are tender and soft, its mind is simple and direct (not complicated and crooked), and it is easy to understand. The simple truth of tai chi—nothing mysterious.

—H. H. Lui

Tai chi is formless form, artless art—fun!

—H. H. Lui

Great squareness has no corners;
Great talents ripen late;
Great music is soft;
Great Form is shapeless.

—Lao Tzu, trans. John C. H. Wu

Tai chi is a poem without words, a song without sound.

—H. H. Lui

Tai chi is the best chi gung.

—H. H. Lui

Tai chi is very tolerant, very flexible.

—H. H. Lui

In quietude, be as still as a mountain; in movement, go like the current of a river.

—Wang Chung-Yueh

The yin yang motion theory:
Everything in the universe is programmed in such a manner that it is continuously contrasting and complementary to itself. This means that everything is continuously showing the negative and positive part of itself.

—H. H. Lui

Tai chi consists of one yin and one yang. The harmonious interplay of yin and yang is Tao. On the Tao, things grow!

—H. H. Lui

Tai chi is a great subtle art of yielding. When the "rock person" pushes the "water person," it just becomes labor lost and frustrating. When you yield, not only the body must yield but also the mind. Then you can adapt.

—H. H. Lui

Heart: a strong dose of Vitamin L (love). Have the heart of a child. No one can enter the world of tai chi without the heart of a child.

Harmony: a sense of being at one within, with others, with nature. Be at peace rather than at war within yourself. Inner conflict is a prime obstacle to tai chi progress. Only harmony within the body and mind can bring tai chi success.

—H. H. Lui

No rice, no energy. No energy, no life.

The universe is chi—full of energy and very lovely. The living body is a universe in miniature and also is chi. The chi of the universe and the chi of the living body are basically of the same nature and the same family.

It is the self (I-center or ego) of the body that blocks the free flowing of the chi between the body and the universe, thus the body becomes isolated, insecure, and weak. Only when you are selfless (tai chi education), can you become an organic part of the universe!

—H. H. Lui

That the weak overcomes the strong, and the
 soft overcomes the hard,
This is something known by all, but practiced
 by none.

—Lao Tzu, trans. John C. H. Wu

The universe is energy and the living body is energy. When the two energies have good communication, you are the universe.

—H. H. Lui

Between heaven and earth, there exists a life force or energy, called chi, which is somewhat like steam to a steamboat. Chi serves to make things move or bounce. It is the chi that makes the tai chi movement light and nimble, change and grow. It is the chi that makes a person feel the sensational fulfillment in doing the exercise. With the absence of chi, there can be no tai chi chuan.

Chi fills the universe. The universe is chi. Thus, it should surprise no one to learn that there is chi flowing through the human mind and body. The better the communication and harmonious oneness a person has with the universe, the more chi with which that person is gifted.

Tai chi is an art of conserving chi. The secret of tai chi is to harmonize ourselves with the movement of the universe and bring ourselves into accord with the universe itself. Thus, tai chi is the work of giving life to all beings and not struggling or competing with each other.

—H. H. Lui

On the tai chi merry-go-round of life,
good-bye means see you again!

—H. H. Lui

EDITOR'S ACKNOWLEDGMENTS

This book was born from curiosity and opportunity. I never studied with Mr. Lui, but heard stories and quotations from those who did, beginning with my first class in 1994. My thanks to Suzanne Roth, my first tai chi teacher, who quoted Lui on tai chi and on life, piquing my interest and curiosity.

My gratitude goes to Judith A. Chambliss whose knowledge and love of all things Lui, and her teaching of same, led me to an active search for Lui sayings and an understanding of Lui's teachings. She and I read through the Lui archives, several boxes of the letters and handouts written by Mr. Lui, sometimes with help from his students. That exploration and opportunity led to the 2004 version of *Spiritual Snacks: Tai Chi to Chew On*, a booklet of quotes based on the archival materials and a series of interviews with people who had studied with Mr. Lui. In 2011, I revised *Spiritual Snacks* to reflect additions and corrections to the text suggested by Mr. Lui's students.

Through the past twenty years, tai chi teachers in the Lui Tai Chi Family have distributed that early booklet to their students, and teachers and students alike have shared it with their friends.

In 2022, Kearns, Howard & Walker suggested it was time for a revised version in book format to offer these teachings to a wider audience. I enthusiastically agreed to provide editorial leadership, with the caveat that *Spiritual Snacks* remain a community effort.

The team that worked with me to renew and revise *Spiritual Snacks* included Karen Ann, Brad Bennett, Jeff Gersten, and Nancy Hoffman. Everyone worked on this project with dedication, thoughtful insight, and commitment. The team provided an overall vision, specific quotations to be included, organization of the book, copyediting, and design.

The *Spiritual Snacks* team extends our deep gratitude to Mr. Lui's former students who readily shared their memories of Mr. Lui's teachings, some back in the booklet days, some more recently:

Donald Beere, Kathleen Brown, James C. Bush, Damian Caspary, Judith A. Chambliss, Patricia Annette Hayford Coen, Christine Durbin, Robert Flannery, Christopher Gentry, Jane Hale, Patrick Johnson, Yofe Johnson, Patricia C. Kearns, Daniel Webster ("Web") Kirksey, Gloria Matuszewski, Nora Privitera, Suzanne Roth, and Allan Bruce Zee.

Our thanks to early readers Kathleen Brown, James C. Bush, Judith A. Chambliss, Ann Link, Peter G. Schmidt, and Allan Bruce Zee.

Our thanks to Gloria Matuszewski for the beautiful cover art.

Barbara Alderson, *Editor*
July 2024

The text of *Spiritual Snacks: Teachings of H. H. Lui* is set in Minion, designed by Robert Slimbach, and titles and pagination are set in Myriad, designed by Robert Slimbach and Carol Twombly.

Printed in March 2025 by Bookmobile Craft Digital in Minneapolis, Minnesota. Inside pages were printed on Lynx® Opaque Ultra 80-lb. white paper produced by Domtar. The cover was printed on Tango® C1S 10 pt. white paper produced by Smurfit WestRock.

KEARNS, HOWARD & WALKER is the publishing arm of the Hubert H. & Elsie Lui Family of Students, originally established in Chicago in 1968 and subsequently based in San Francisco and the Bay Area from 1979 to the present. Based in the states of California, New York, Oregon, Virginia, and Washington | United States of America

www.khwpublisher.com